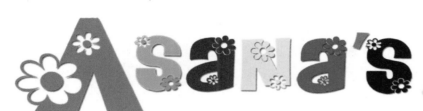

Asana's Yoga Class

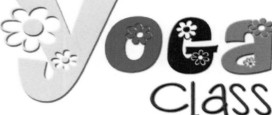

Namaste'

ARE YOU READY TO DO YOGA WITH ME?

I am active

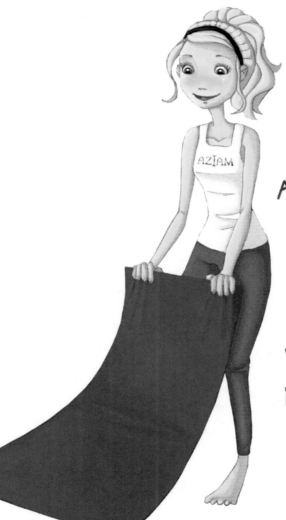

WRitten by Alanna Zabel

illustRated by Rita Vigovszky

Published by AZIAM Books.
© 2013 Alanna Zabel.
All rights reserved.

ISBN-13: 978-0-9862075-0-1

AZIAM Books
Santa Monica, CA
www.aziam.com

AZ|AM
BOOKS

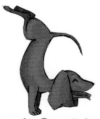

Dedicated to the mental and phyisical
Health & Fitness of our Youth.

10% of book sale Profits benefit:
Alliance For A Healthier Generation

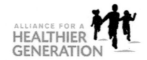

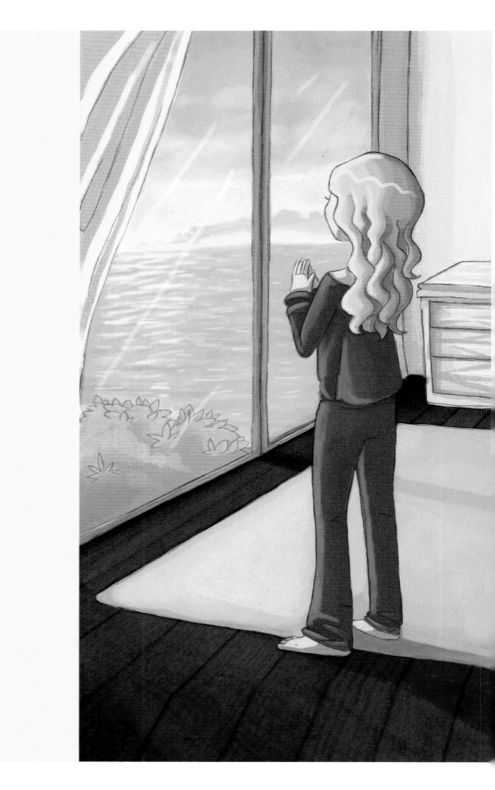

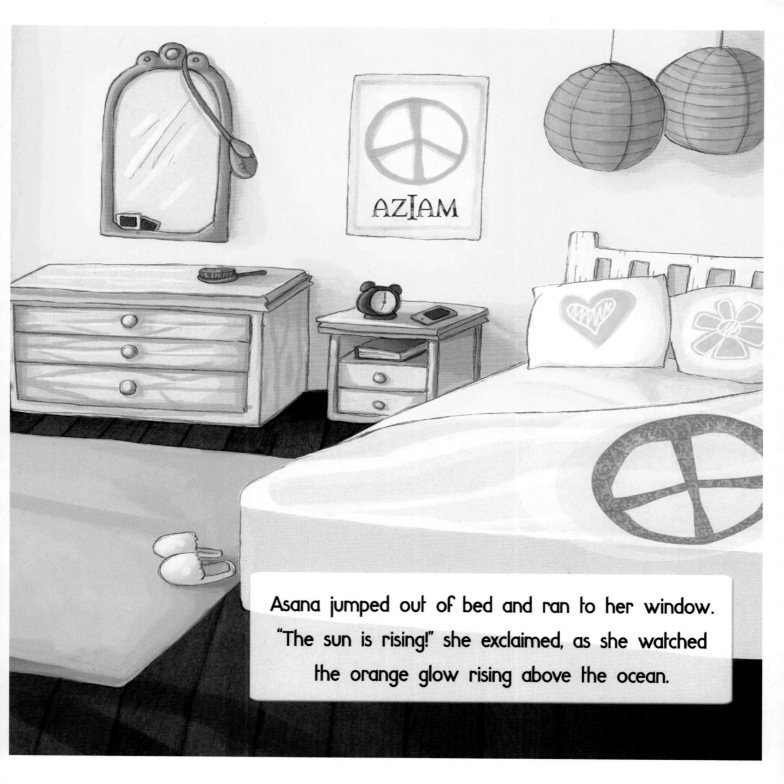

Asana jumped out of bed and ran to her window. "The sun is rising!" she exclaimed, as she watched the orange glow rising above the ocean.

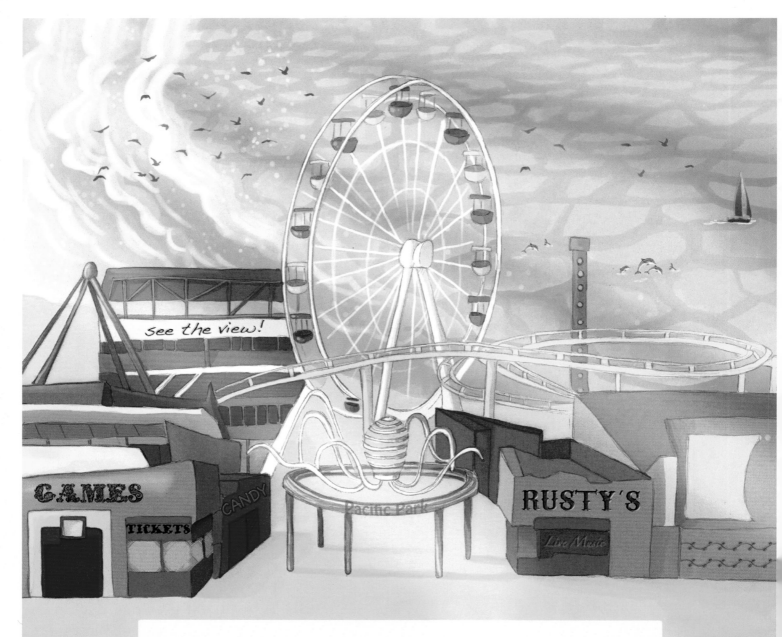

The ferris wheel on the Santa Monica Pier glistened
in the sunlight, while flocks of birds and schools
of dolphins celebrated the new morning..

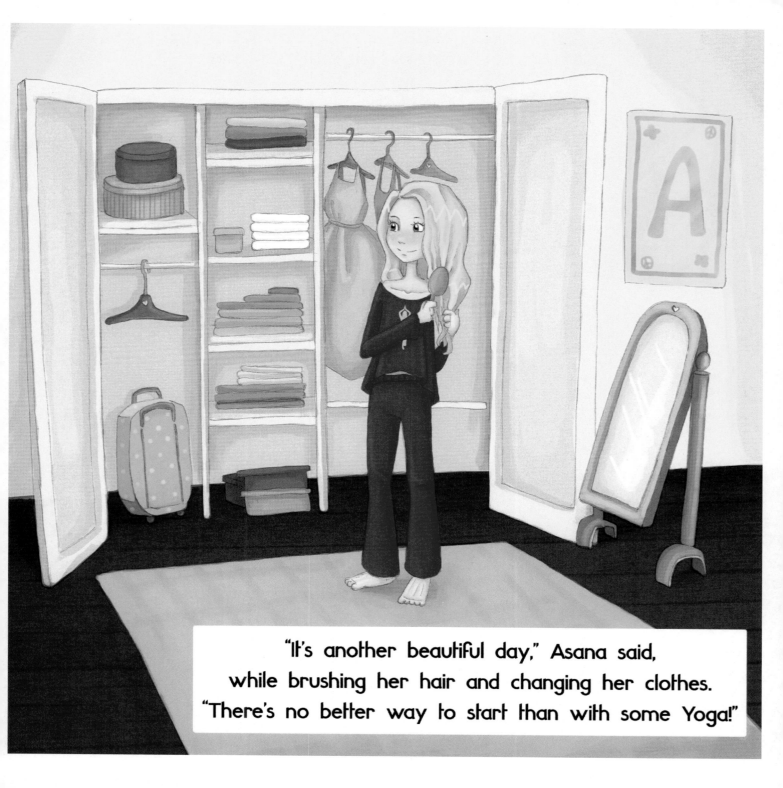

"It's another beautiful day," Asana said,
while brushing her hair and changing her clothes.
"There's no better way to start than with some Yoga!"

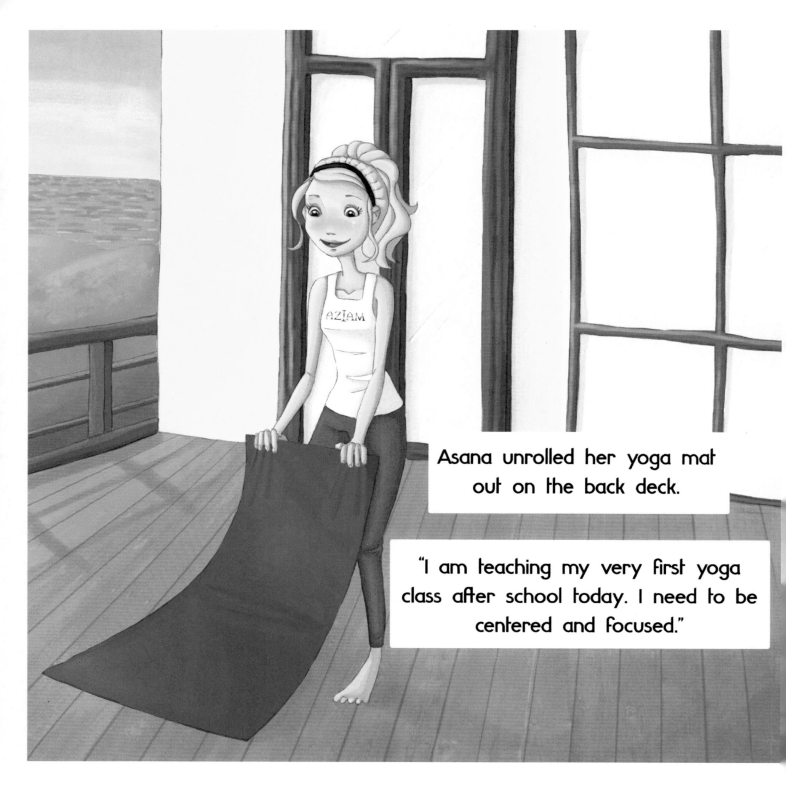

Asana unrolled her yoga mat out on the back deck.

"I am teaching my very first yoga class after school today. I need to be centered and focused."

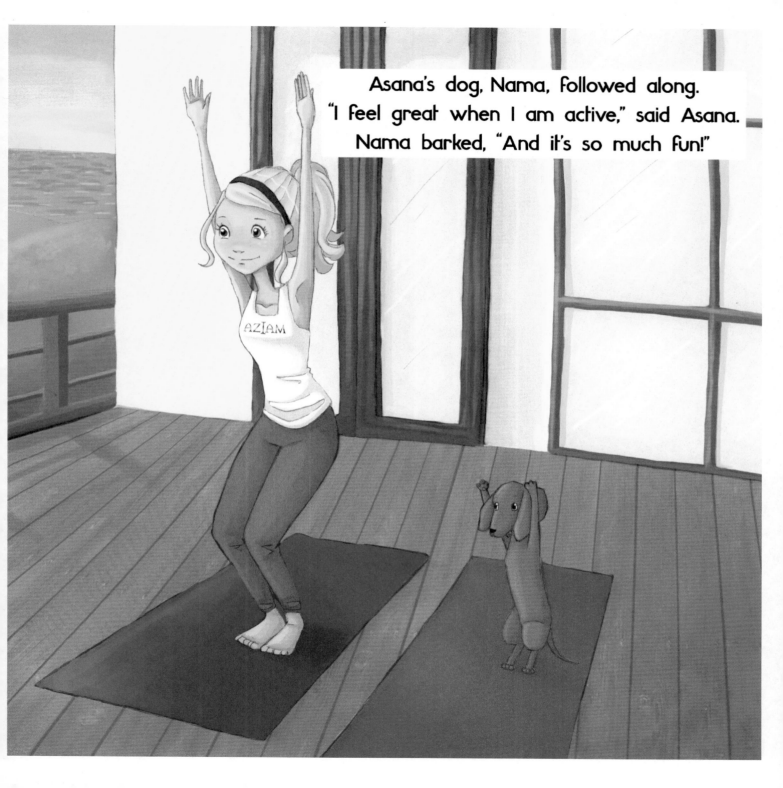

Asana's dog, Nama, followed along.
"I feel great when I am active," said Asana.
Nama barked, "And it's so much fun!"

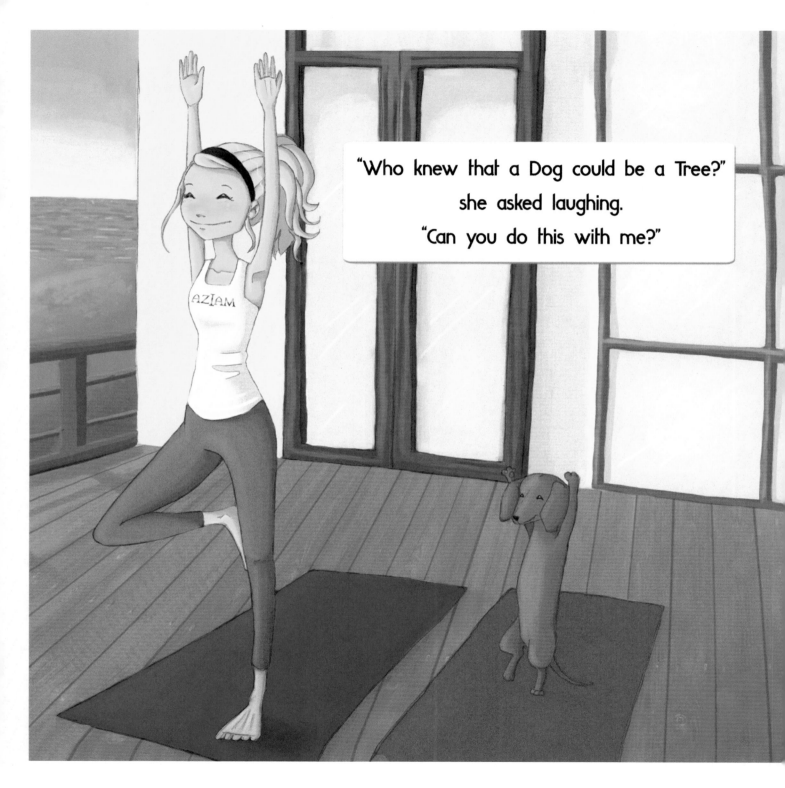

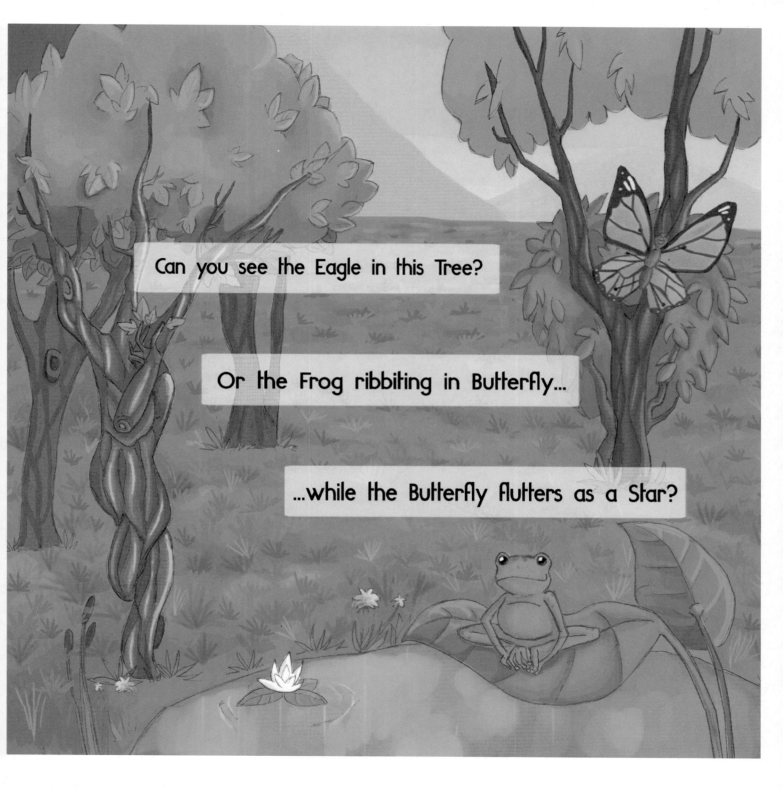

Can you see the Eagle in this Tree?

Or the Frog ribbiting in Butterfly...

...while the Butterfly flutters as a Star?

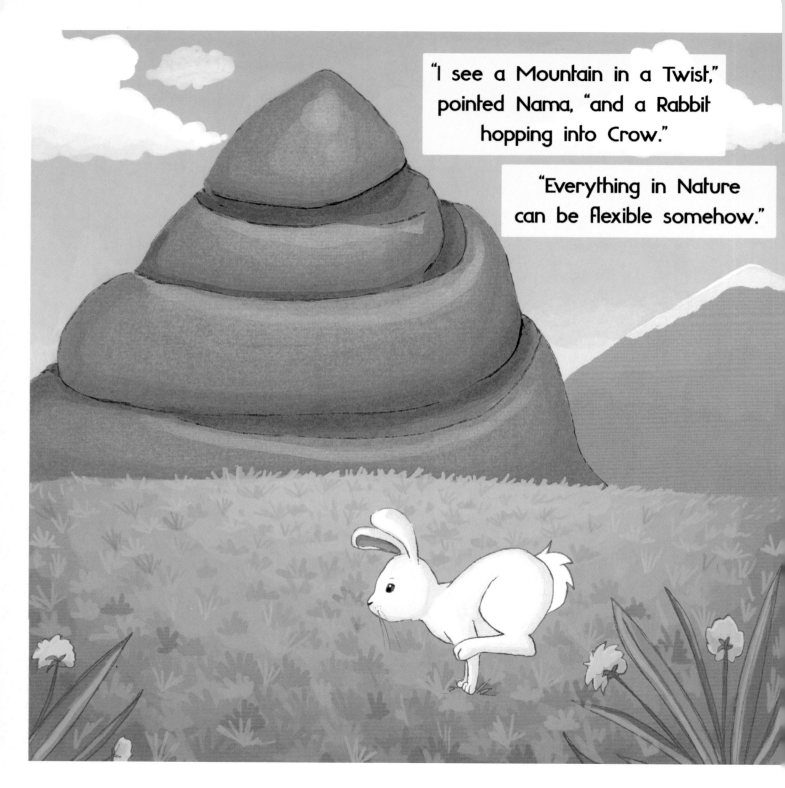

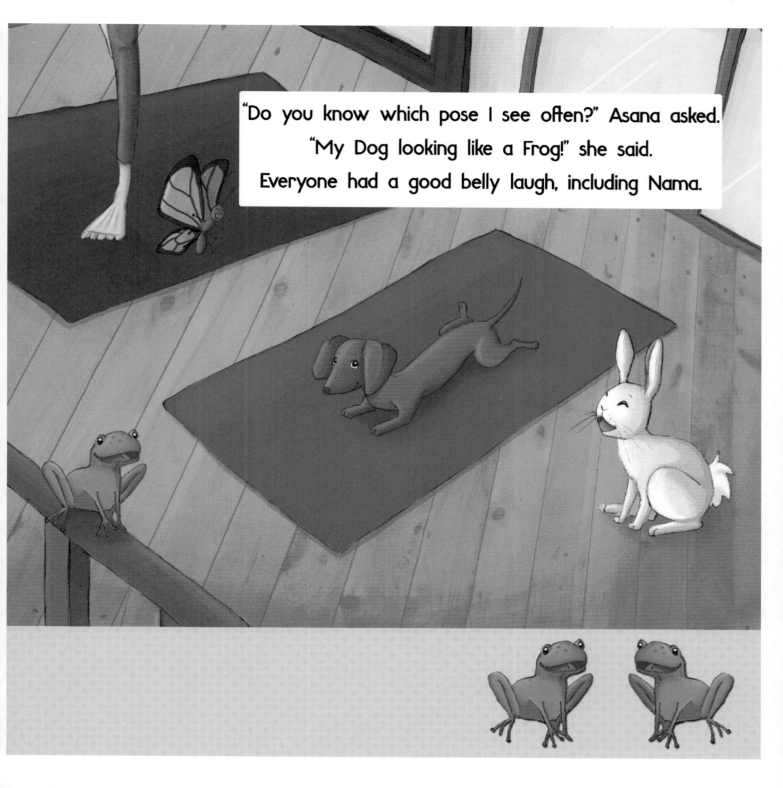

"Do you know which pose I see often?" Asana asked.

"My Dog looking like a Frog!" she said.

Everyone had a good belly laugh, including Nama.

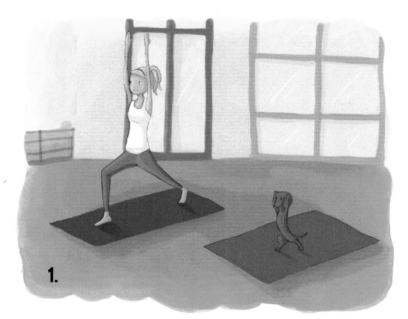

1.

Asana and Nama practiced their Sun
Salutations, moving through Warrior 1
and Warrior 2 into Warrior 3.

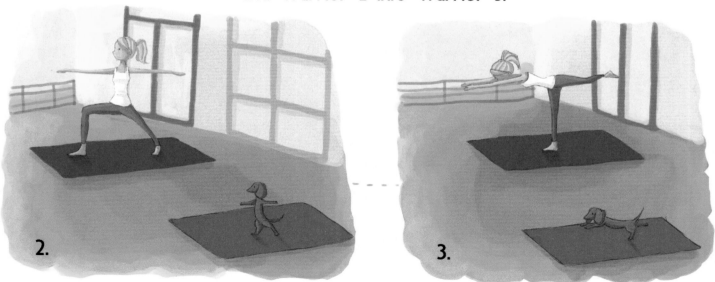

2.

3.

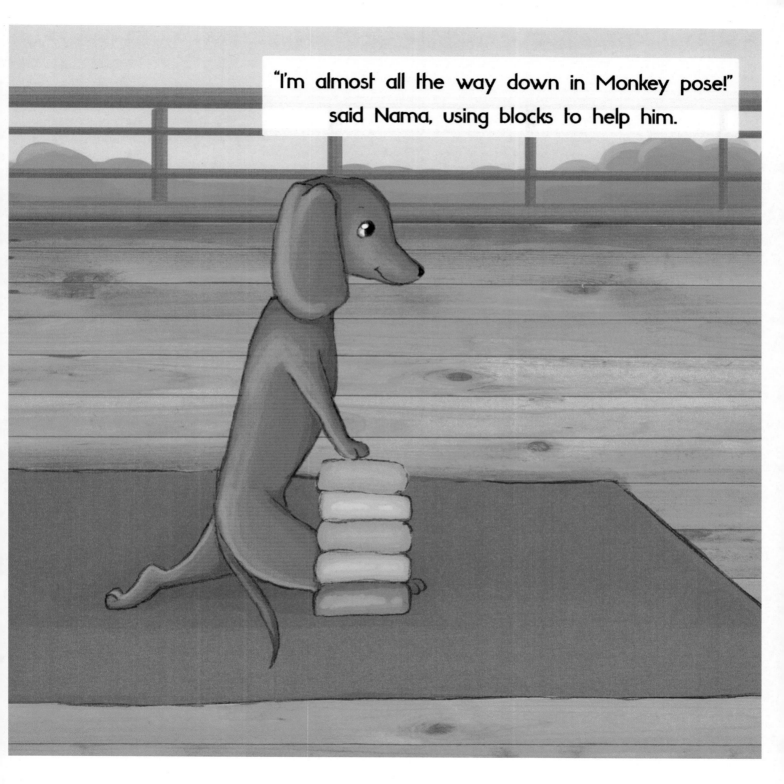

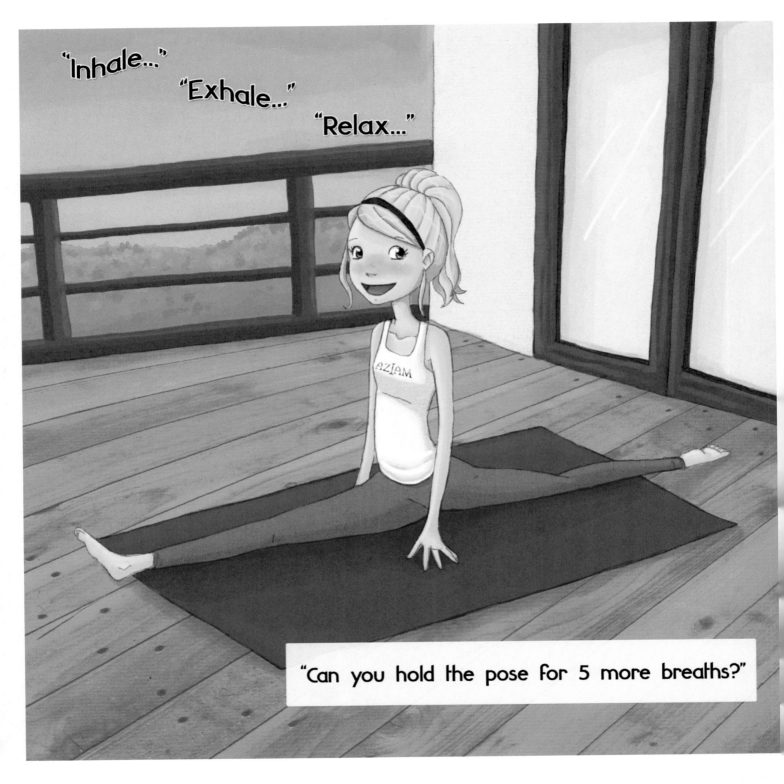

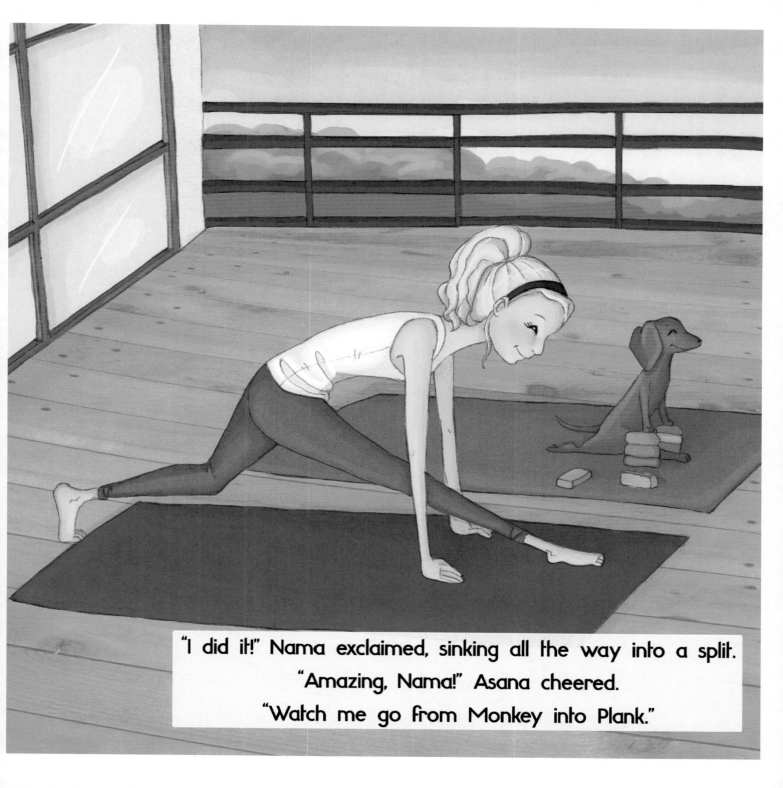

"I did it!" Nama exclaimed, sinking all the way into a split.
"Amazing, Nama!" Asana cheered.
"Watch me go from Monkey into Plank."

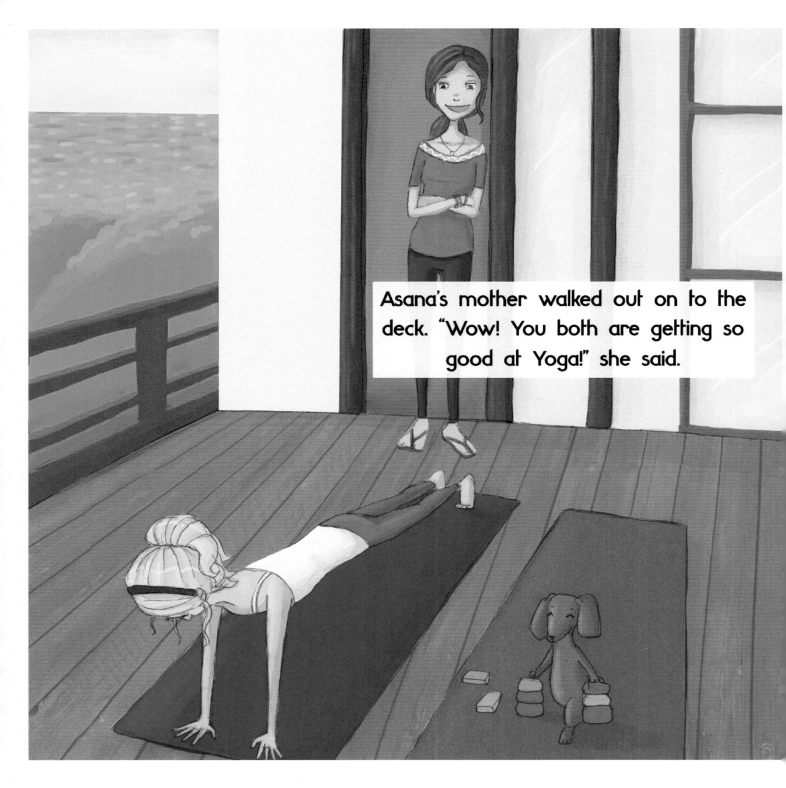

Asana's mother walked out on to the deck. "Wow! You both are getting so good at Yoga!" she said.

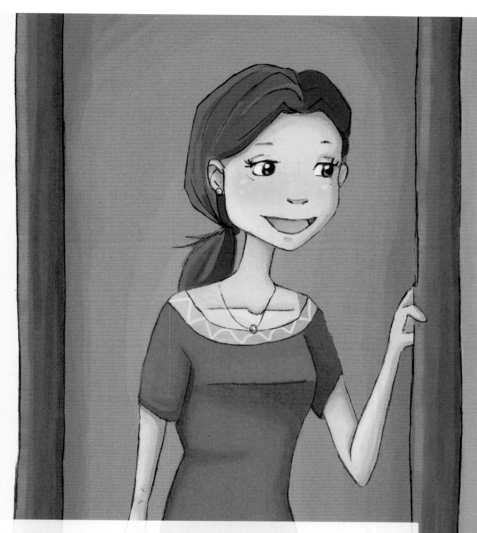

"But Darling, you need to get ready for school so that you won't be late," her Mom continued.

"You have a really big day. All of the A.Z.I.AM Girlz will be here after school to take your yoga class."

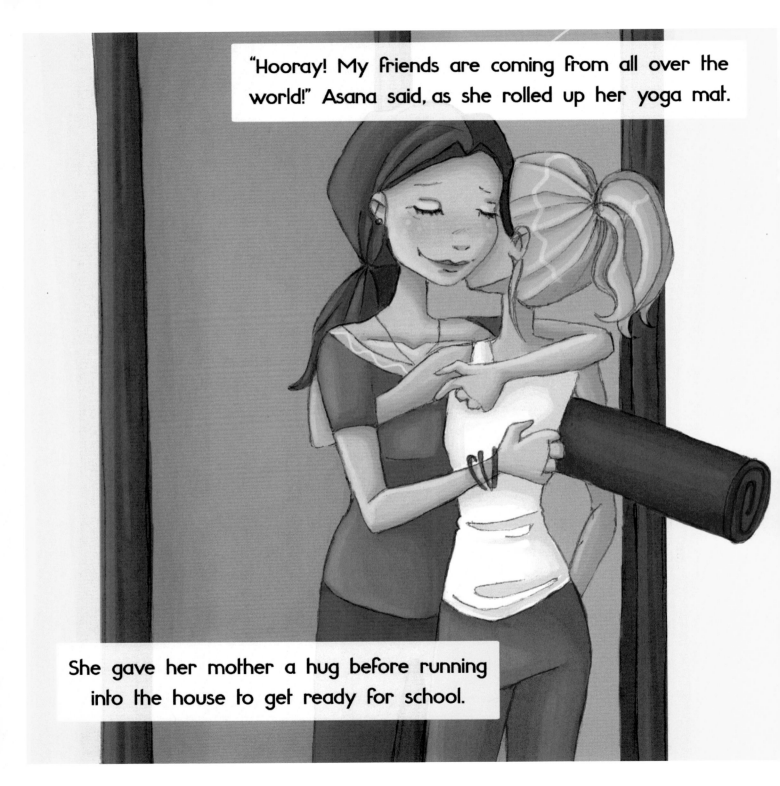

"Hooray! My friends are coming from all over the world!" Asana said, as she rolled up her yoga mat.

She gave her mother a hug before running into the house to get ready for school.

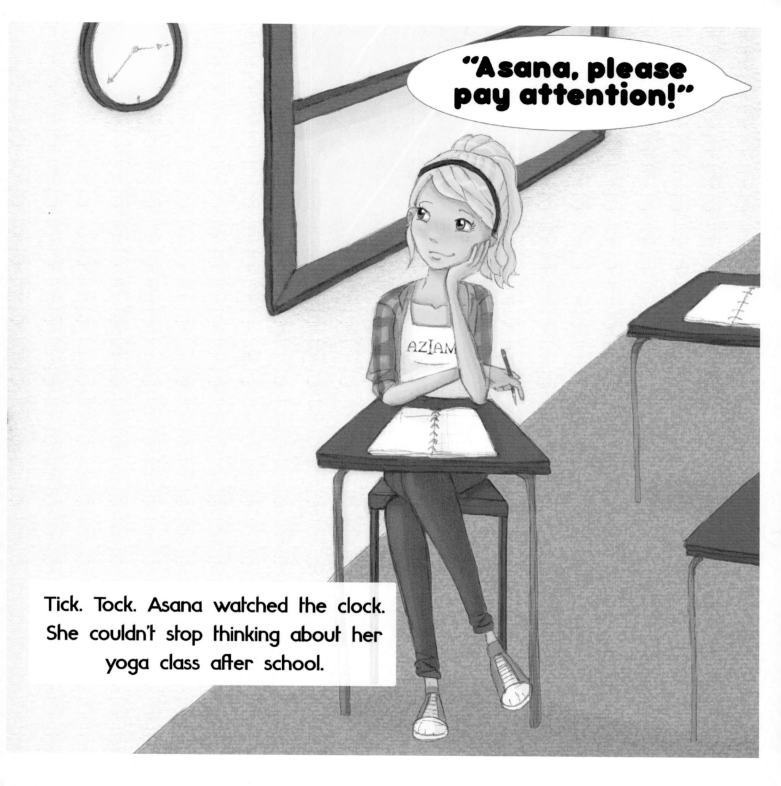

"Asana, please pay attention!"

Tick. Tock. Asana watched the clock. She couldn't stop thinking about her yoga class after school.

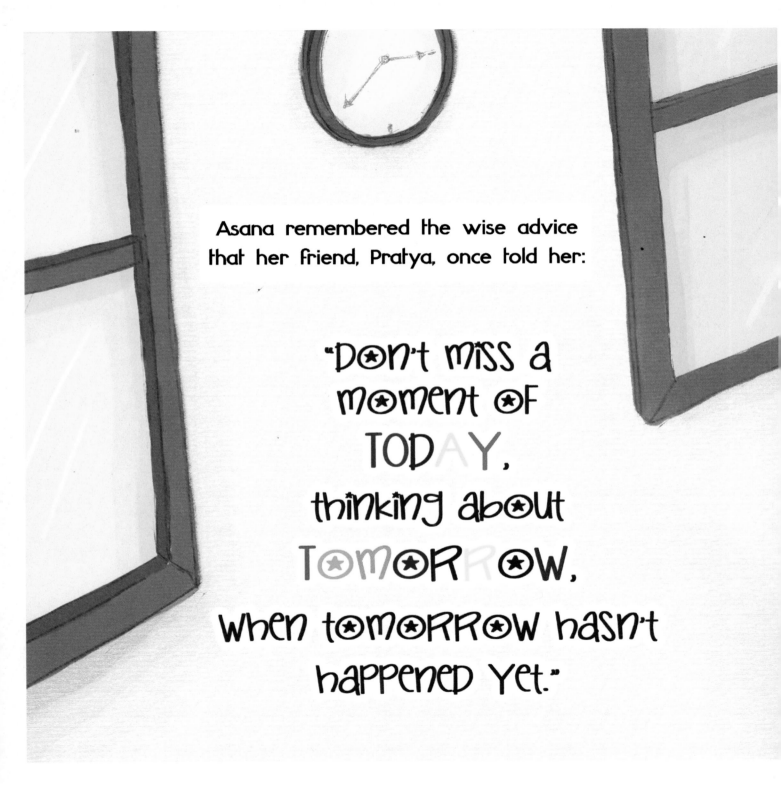

Asana remembered the wise advice that her friend, Pratya, once told her:

"Don't miss a moment of TODAY, thinking about TOMORROW, when tomorrow hasn't happened yet."

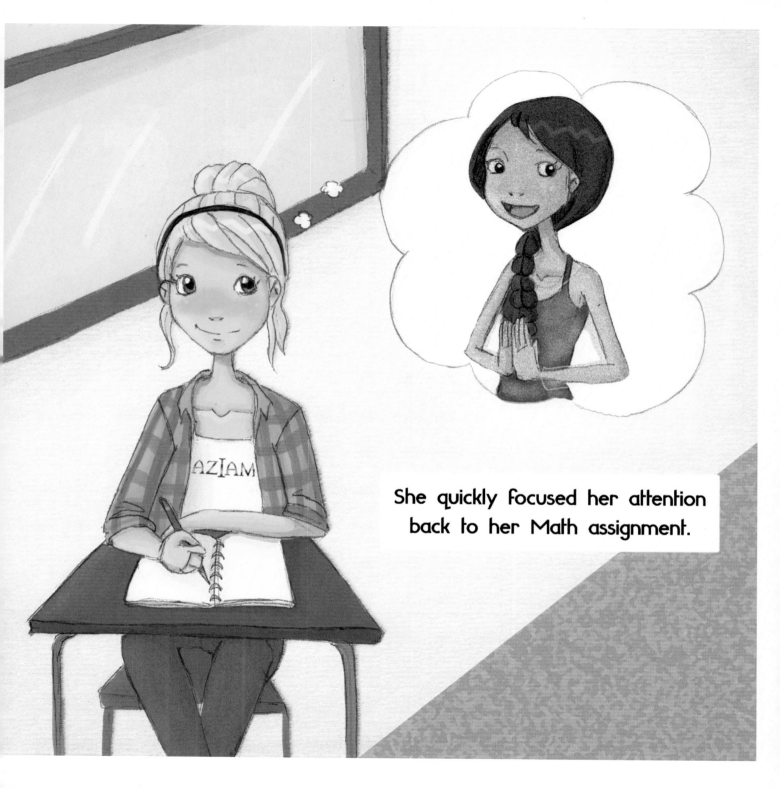

She quickly focused her attention back to her Math assignment.

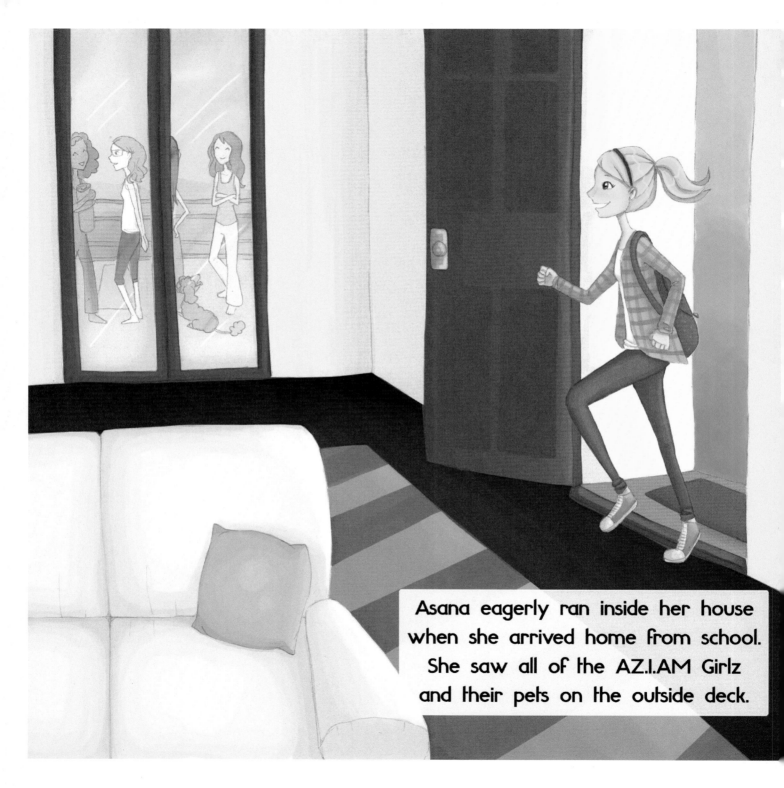

Asana eagerly ran inside her house when she arrived home from school. She saw all of the AZ.I.AM Girlz and their pets on the outside deck.

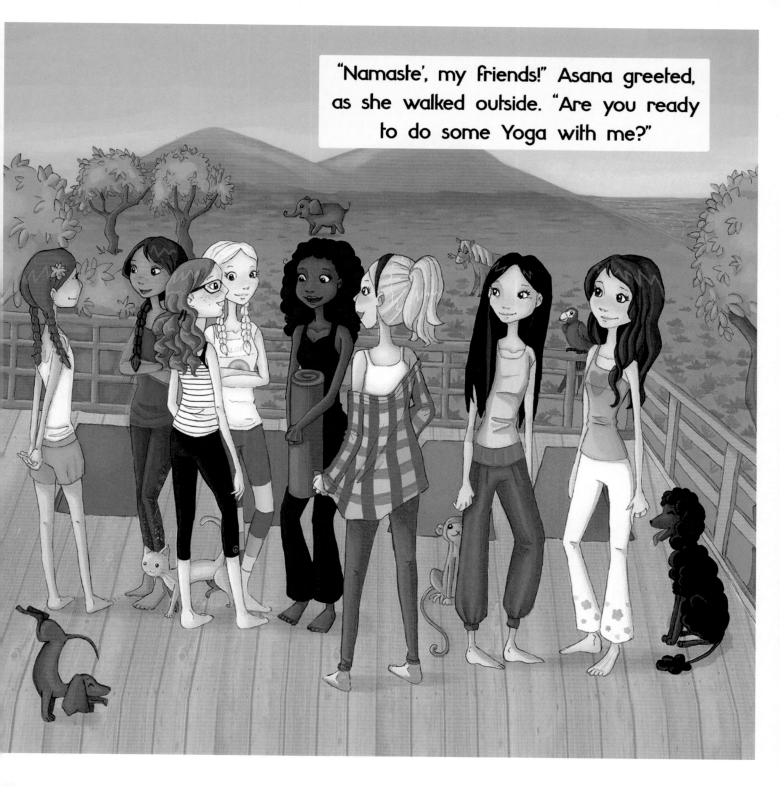

"Namaste', my friends!" Asana greeted, as she walked outside. "Are you ready to do some Yoga with me?"

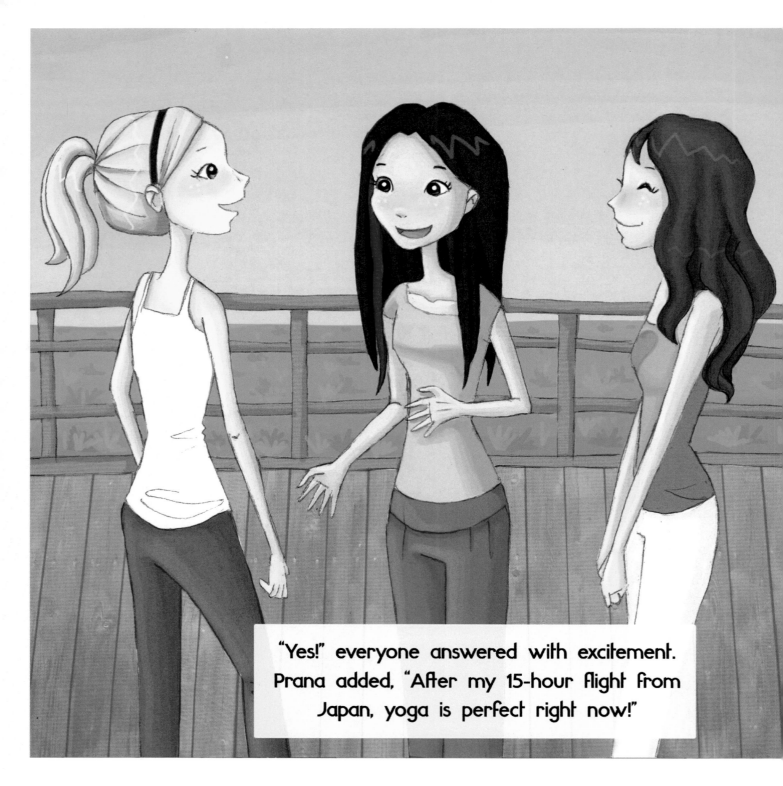

"Yes!" everyone answered with excitement. Prana added, "After my 15-hour flight from Japan, yoga is perfect right now!"

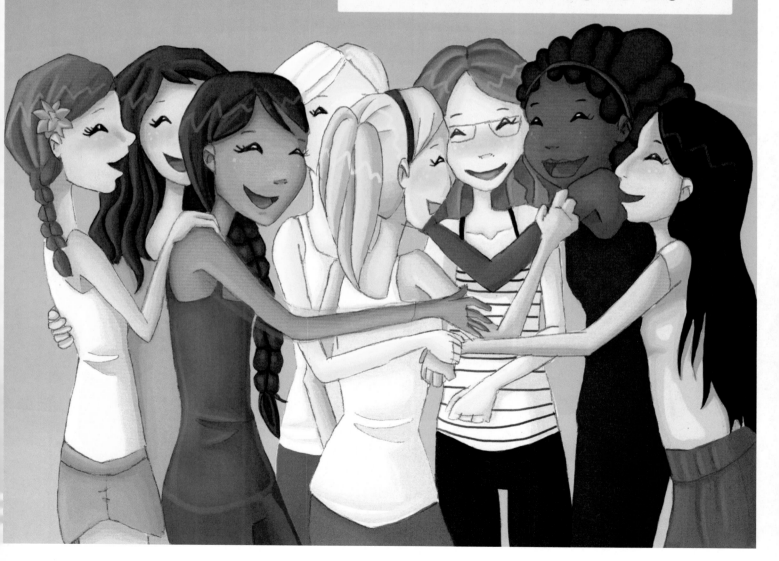

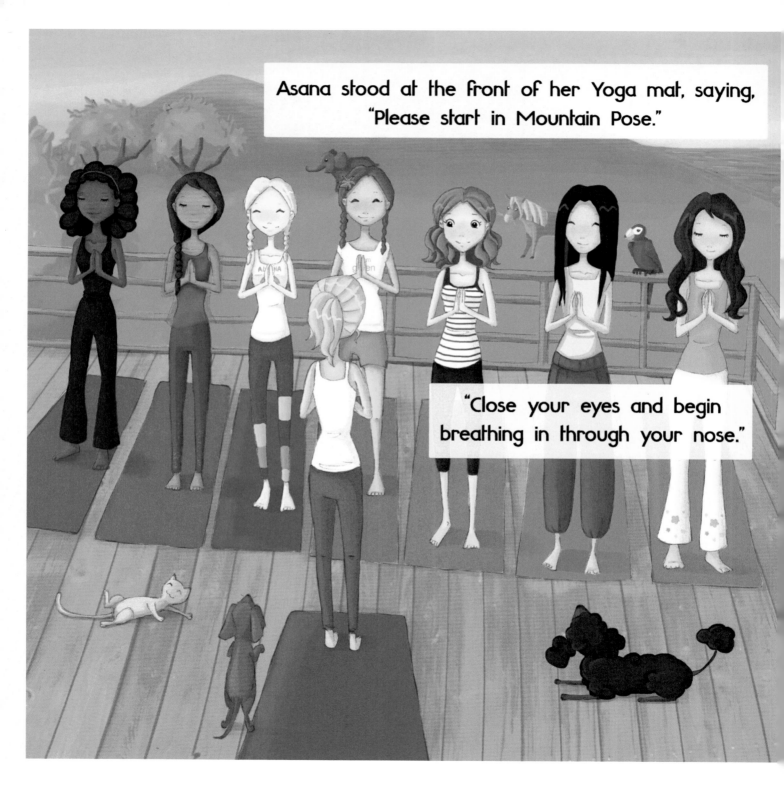

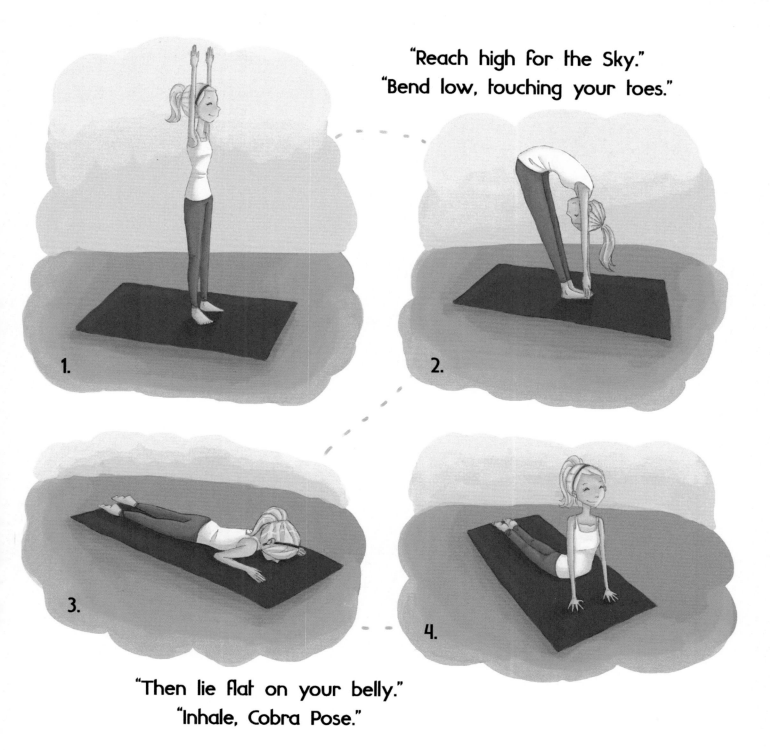

"Reach high for the Sky."
"Bend low, touching your toes."

"Then lie flat on your belly."
"Inhale, Cobra Pose."

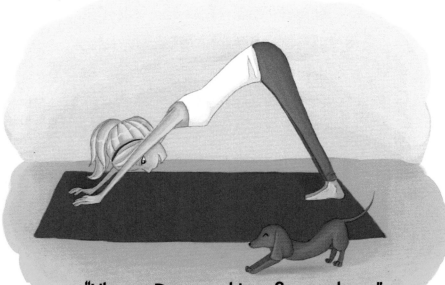

"Like a Dog waking from sleep,"
"Stretch your legs and back, too."

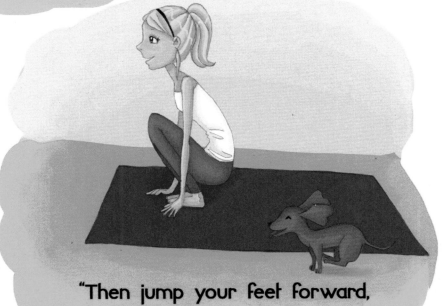

"Then jump your feet forward,
like a happy Kanagroo!"

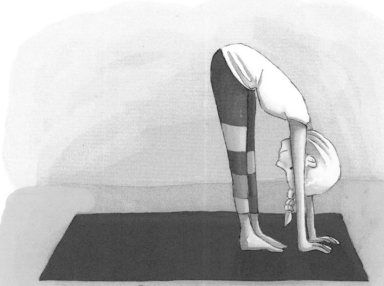

"Yoga really makes you strong,"
said Yama.

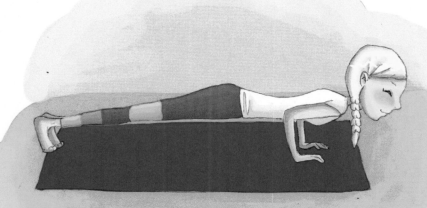

As she jumped back from Earth Pose to
to Grasshopper (or Chattaranga).

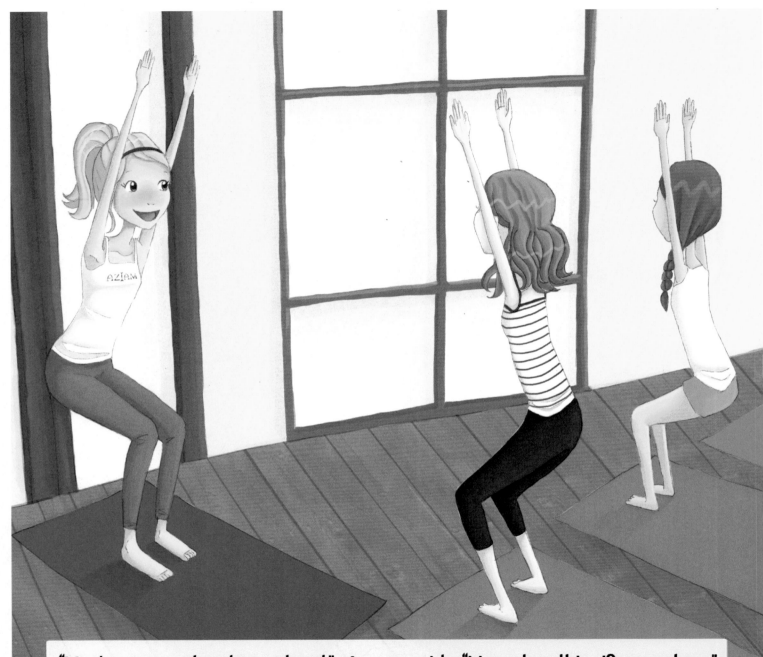

"You're a spectacular natural," Asana said,. "Now try this, if you dare."
"Bend your knees, and have a seat on a Chair in the air."

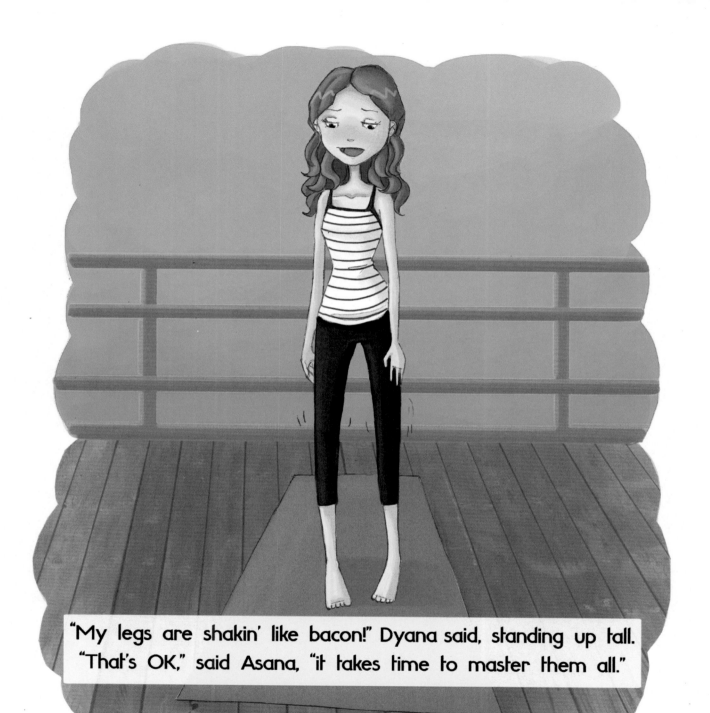

"My legs are shakin' like bacon!" Dyana said, standing up tall.
"That's OK," said Asana, "it takes time to master them all."

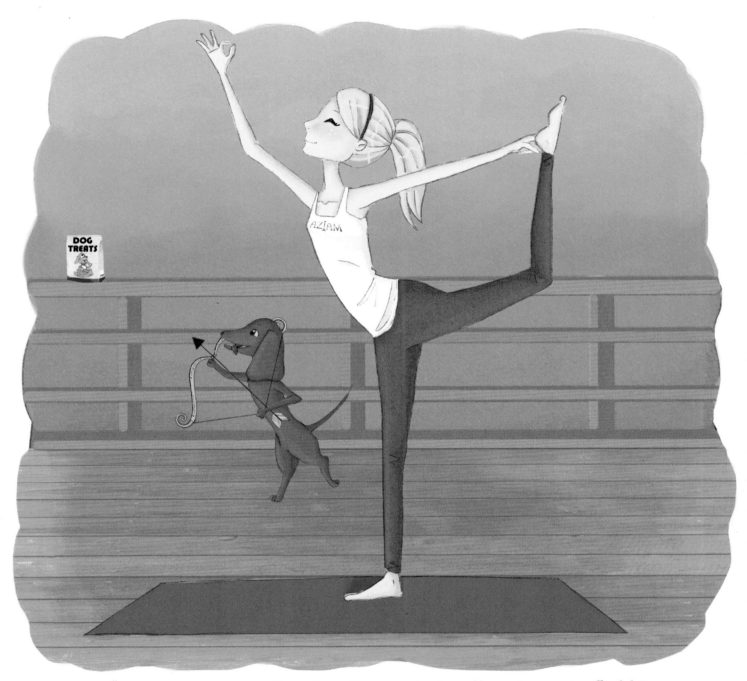

"Here we go, a Standing Bow, aiming the Arrow's flight."
"Balance and Focus. Five breaths left, and five breaths right."

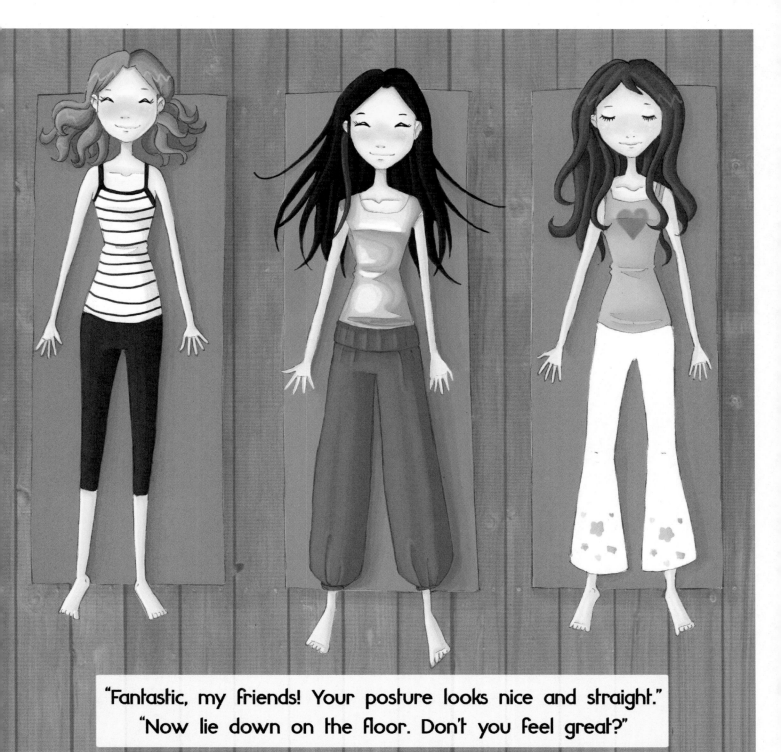

"Fantastic, my friends! Your posture looks nice and straight."
"Now lie down on the floor. Don't you feel great?"

"Swing your legs over your head, like a Plow in the field."
"When you take care of your body, you help it to heal."

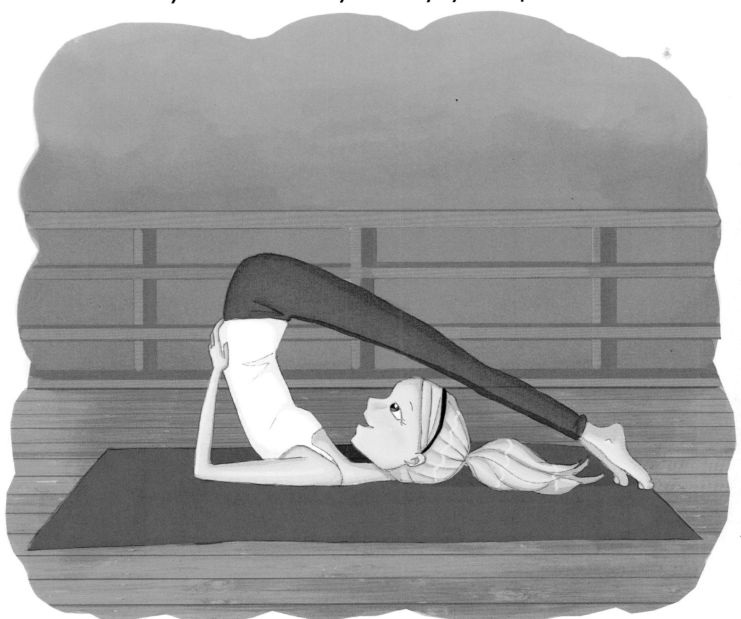

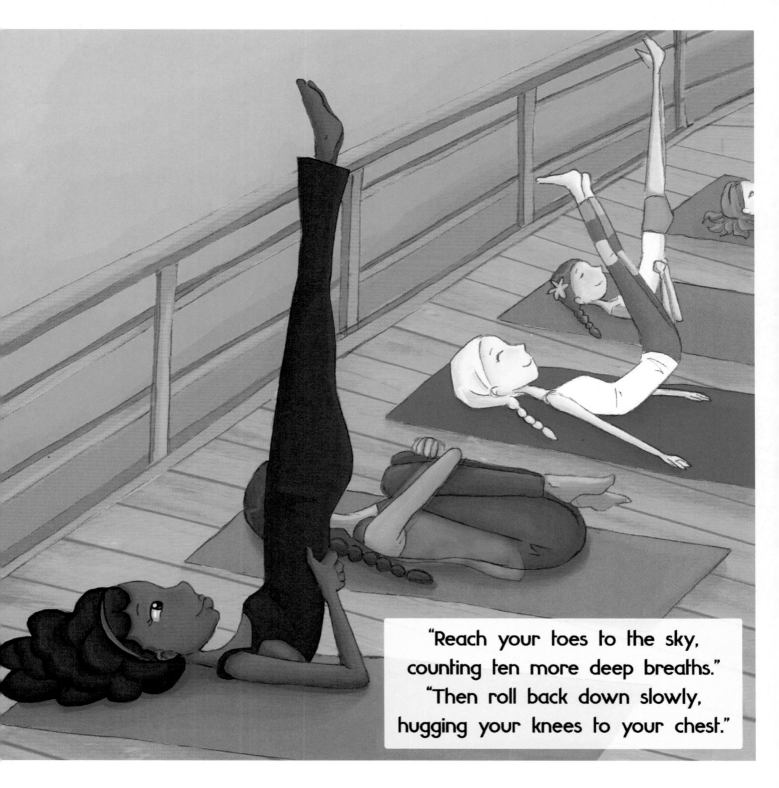

"Reach your toes to the sky, counting ten more deep breaths." "Then roll back down slowly, hugging your knees to your chest."

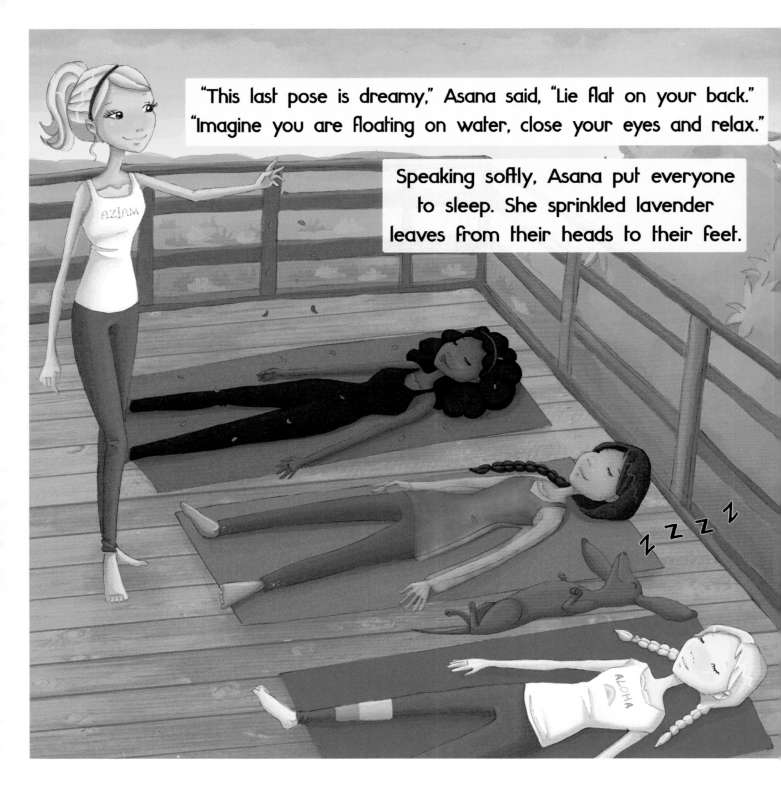

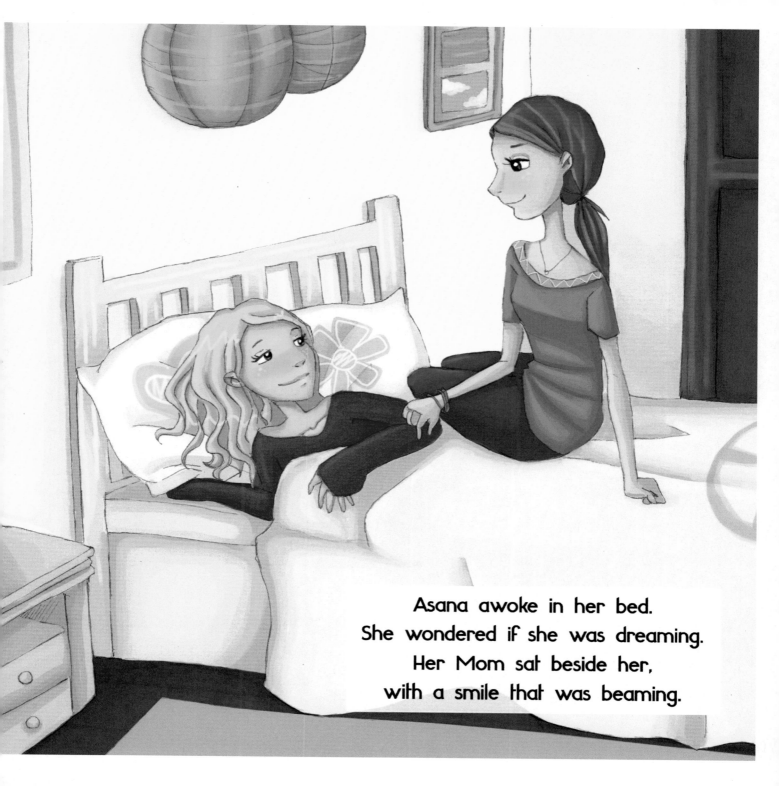

Asana awoke in her bed.
She wondered if she was dreaming.
Her Mom sat beside her,
with a smile that was beaming.

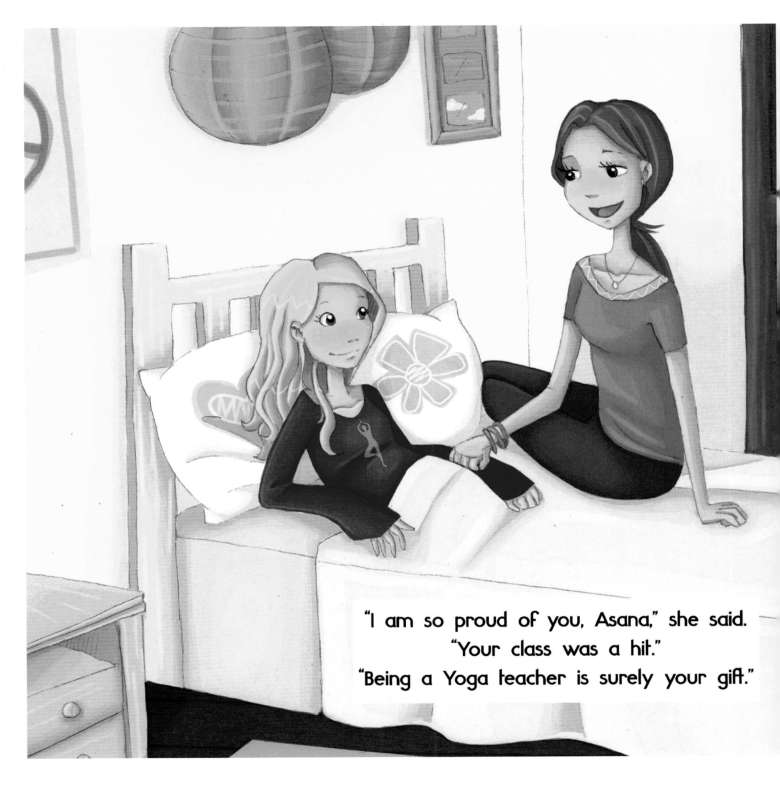

"I am so proud of you, Asana," she said.
"Your class was a hit."
"Being a Yoga teacher is surely your gift."

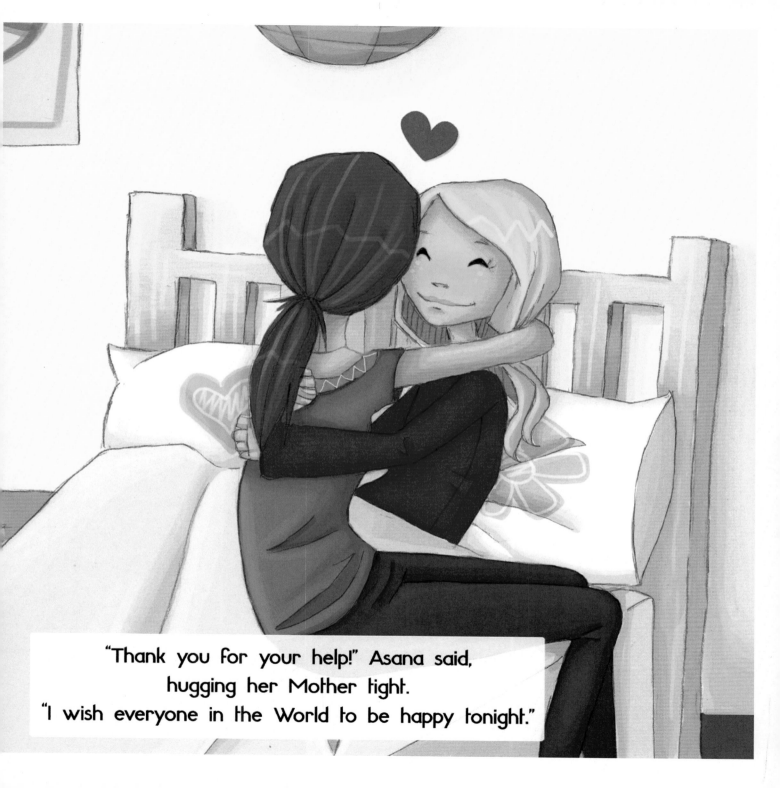

"Thank you for your help!" Asana said,
hugging her Mother tight.
"I wish everyone in the World to be happy tonight."

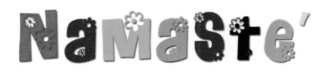

The Light Within Me
Sees the Light Within YOU

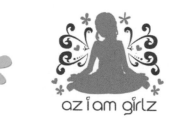

az i am girlz

i am a GiRL who wants to see WORLD peace

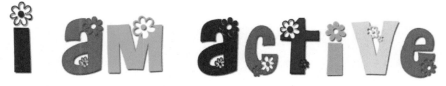

i am active

i am Healthy
i am kind
i am HAPPY
i am Beautiful, exactly az.i.am

Made in the USA
San Bernardino, CA
14 March 2016